The Kidney Disease Lifeline

Empowering Your Journey Through Understanding, Treatment, and Holistic Care for Improved Health and Quality of Life

Tricia Whitner

Table of Contents

Chapter Four: Living with Kidney Disease 69

PREFACE

As a Nephrologist, I have spent countless hours in the clinic and hospital settings, witnessing firsthand the challenges and struggles faced by individuals battling kidney disease. From the initial shock of diagnosis to the complexities of management and treatment, the journey with kidney disease is often fraught with uncertainty, fear, and numerous questions. It is a journey that affects not just the physical body but also the emotional and psychological well-being of patients and their families.

My motivation to write this book stems from a deep desire to extend the reach of my support beyond the confines of my office, to touch the lives of those I may never meet in person. I hope to bridge the gap between the clinical encounters and the day-to-day realities of living with kidney disease, providing a resource that is not only informative but also empathetic and empowering.

In these pages, I aim to demystify kidney disease, breaking down the complexities of renal function, the mechanisms behind the disease, and the rationale for various treatment options into understandable language. My goal is to offer a guide that illuminates the path through diagnosis, management, and beyond, equipping you with the knowledge to make informed decisions about your care and to advocate for your health with confidence.

Moreover, this book is an invitation to see beyond the disease. It is a call to embrace a lifestyle that supports kidney health, to recognize the power of a supportive community, and to find strength in the face of adversity. I share insights into navigating the healthcare system, managing the financial impact of chronic illness, and maintaining quality of life despite the challenges posed by kidney disease.

To my readers, know that you are not alone on this journey. Through these pages, I hope to offer you companionship, guidance, and hope. Whether you are newly diagnosed, a caregiver, or someone looking to deepen your understanding of kidney disease, this book is for you. Together, let us embark on this journey towards better health, armed with knowledge, empowered by understanding, and united in hope.

With warm regards,

Tricia Whitner.

INTRODUCTION

The human body is a marvel of nature, a complex system where each part has a role crucial for overall health and well-being. At the heart of this system, functioning quietly yet indispensably, are the kidneys. These bean-shaped organs, each about the size of a fist, are located just below the rib cage on either side of the spine. Despite their modest size, kidneys are mighty workers, performing several vital functions essential to maintaining life. They filter and remove waste products and excess fluids from the blood through urine, regulate blood pressure, balance electrolytes, and produce hormones critical for red blood cell production and bone health.

However, when the kidneys do not perform their functions properly due to damage or disease, the consequences for the body can be severe. Kidney disease, in its various forms, represents a significant and growing challenge to public health worldwide. It is a condition where the kidneys are damaged and cannot filter blood as well as they should. This damage can accumulate over time and may lead to kidney failure, a life-threatening condition requiring dialysis or a kidney transplant.

The insidious nature of kidney disease is that it can develop with few symptoms in its early stages. Many people are unaware they have kidney disease until it has progressed. Early signs, such as fatigue, swollen ankles, and changes in urine output, are often overlooked or attributed to less serious health issues. This lack of awareness underscores the critical importance of early diagnosis. Detecting kidney disease in its nascent stages can significantly slow its progression, prevent complications, and improve outcomes. Routine screenings are especially crucial for those at higher risk, including individuals with diabetes, hypertension, a family history of kidney disease, and certain ethnic groups.

Early intervention, based on a timely diagnosis, can dramatically alter the disease's trajectory. It can involve lifestyle changes, dietary adjustments, medication to control symptoms and underlying causes, and regular monitoring of kidney function. Recognizing the early signs and symptoms of kidney disease and understanding the risk factors are the first steps in preventing or delaying the progression of this silent disease.

This book is born out of a commitment to inform, assist, and empower you, the reader, who may be navigating the challenging waters of kidney disease. Whether you are a patient, a caregiver, or someone interested in understanding more about kidney health, this guide is for you. It is designed to demystify the complexities surrounding kidney disease, offering clear, accessible explanations of how the kidneys work, what happens when they don't, and the implications for your health and lifestyle.

Beyond a mere compilation of medical facts, this book aims to be a companion on your journey with kidney disease. It will guide you through understanding the disease's nuances, from diagnosis to treatment options, managing symptoms, and making informed decisions about your care. It seeks to empower you with knowledge, giving you the tools to actively participate in your treatment and advocate for your health.

You can expect to find practical advice on managing kidney disease through dietary and lifestyle changes, insights into the medical treatments available, and tips for living a fulfilling life despite the challenges posed by the condition. This book also addresses the emotional and psychological aspects of dealing with a chronic illness, offering strategies for finding support and maintaining mental well-being.

In writing this book, my goal is to bridge the gap between the clinical information provided in a doctor's office and the real-life implications of living with kidney disease. It is to provide a source of reliable, comprehensive information that can answer your questions, alleviate your fears, and inspire you to take control of your health.

Kidney disease, with its complexities and challenges, can be a daunting prospect for anyone. However, armed with the right information, support, and resources, navigating this condition becomes a journey of empowerment. Through the pages of this book, you will gain not just knowledge but also the confidence to manage your kidney health proactively. Together, we will explore the essential aspects of kidney disease, from the fundamentals of kidney function to the latest in treatment options, all aimed at helping you lead a healthier, more informed life.

CHAPTER ONE: UNDERSTANDING KIDNEY DISEASE

Kidney disease, a silent yet formidable adversary, undermines the health of millions globally. This chapter delves into the essence of kidney disease—its definition, underlying causes, and the stages it encompasses. We navigate through the crucial diagnostic tests that unveil its presence and address the myths clouding its understanding. Our journey through these pages aims to illuminate the complexities of kidney disease, offering clarity and dispelling misconceptions,

What is Kidney Disease?

Kidney disease, often a silent health issue, significantly impacts millions of individuals worldwide, affecting the body's ability to perform its crucial detoxifying functions. The kidneys, two bean-shaped organs located on either side of the spine, below the rib cage, play a pivotal role in maintaining overall health. They are responsible for filtering waste products and excess fluids from the blood, which are then excreted through urine. Beyond waste removal, kidneys are vital in regulating blood pressure, ensuring electrolyte balance, and stimulating the production of red blood cells by releasing erythropoietin. Their health and functionality are, therefore, integral to the body's well-being.

Kidney disease manifests in two primary forms: Chronic and Acute. Chronic Kidney Disease (CKD) involves a slow deterioration of the kidneys' abilities, persisting over an extended period. It is often a consequence of underlying illnesses such as diabetes or high blood pressure, which slowly damage the kidneys and diminish their ability to filter blood effectively. The damage is insidious and can progress to end-stage renal disease (ESRD), where the kidneys fail to work at a level needed for day-to-day life, potentially requiring dialysis or kidney transplantation.

Acute Kidney Injury (AKI), on the other hand, occurs suddenly, often triggered by an injury, severe infection, or certain medications that can cause the kidneys to become inflamed or severely damaged in a short period. Unlike CKD, AKI can be reversible if treated promptly and appropriately, allowing the kidneys to recover their filtering capabilities.

The causes of kidney disease are varied, including genetic predispositions, environmental factors, and chronic conditions like diabetes and hypertension. Diabetes leads to high blood sugar levels that can damage the nephrons, the filtering units of the kidneys, while hypertension can cause damage to the blood vessels in the kidneys, impairing their filtering ability. Other risk factors include obesity, smoking, age, and a family history of kidney disease, which can increase an individual's likelihood of developing kidney issues.

The effects of kidney disease on the body are profound and far-reaching. As kidney function declines, waste products and fluids can accumulate in the body, leading to complications such as high blood pressure, anemia, weak bones, poor nutritional health, and nerve damage. Kidney disease also increases the risk of developing cardiovascular diseases, including heart attacks and strokes, further emphasizing the importance of early detection and management.

Understanding kidney disease's implications is crucial for managing its progression and mitigating its impact on health. Knowledge of the types, causes, and effects of kidney disease lays the foundation for exploring diagnostic methods, treatment options, and strategies for living with the condition, all aimed at preserving kidney health and maintaining quality of life.

Causes and Risk Factors

Kidney disease can stem from a variety of causes and risk factors, ranging from chronic health conditions to lifestyle choices and genetic predispositions. Understanding these can help in assessing risk and taking proactive steps toward prevention.

Chronic Health Conditions

Diabetes is a leading cause of kidney disease. High blood sugar levels, characteristic of diabetes, can damage the blood vessels in the kidneys over time. This damage prevents the kidneys from filtering waste from the blood efficiently, leading to diabetic nephropathy. Managing blood sugar levels through diet, medication, and lifestyle changes is crucial for diabetes patients to lower their risk of developing kidney disease.

Elevated blood pressure (hypertension) is also a major risk contributor. The kidneys use blood pressure to filter blood and remove waste and excess fluids. However, uncontrolled high blood pressure can damage the blood vessels in the kidneys, reducing their ability to function properly. Controlling blood pressure with medication and lifestyle modifications, such as reducing salt intake and regular physical activity, is vital.

Genetic Predispositions

Certain kidney diseases can be hereditary, passed down from one generation to another. Polycystic kidney disease (PKD), for example, is a genetic disorder characterized by the growth of numerous cysts in the kidneys, which can interfere with kidney function and lead to CKD. A family history of CKD or other kidney diseases significantly increases an individual's risk, highlighting the importance of genetic counseling and regular screenings for those with a family history of kidney conditions.

Environmental or Lifestyle Factors

Lifestyle choices play a significant role in the development of kidney disease. Obesity, for instance, can lead to diabetes and hypertension, both of which are risk factors for kidney disease. A diet high in sodium and processed foods can increase blood pressure, while smoking can damage blood vessels, including those in the kidneys, impairing their function.

Environmental factors, such as exposure to certain chemicals and pollutants, can also contribute to the risk of developing kidney disease. Some substances, including heavy metals like lead and mercury, can accumulate in the kidneys and cause damage. Occupations that expose individuals to such chemicals should enforce protective measures to minimize risk.

Assessing Risk and Prevention

Understanding personal risk factors is the first step in preventing kidney disease. Individuals with a family history of kidney disease, those suffering from diabetes, hypertension, or obesity, and smokers are at higher risk and should consider regular kidney function screenings. Prevention strategies include maintaining a healthy weight, adopting a balanced diet low in sodium, managing chronic conditions like diabetes and hypertension, regular exercise, and avoiding tobacco and excessive alcohol use.

Regular check-ups with healthcare providers can help in early detection and management of conditions that may lead to kidney disease. For those at higher risk, monitoring blood pressure, blood sugar levels, and kidney function through periodic tests can be crucial in preventing kidney damage or catching it early when it is most treatable.

By understanding the causes and risk factors of kidney disease and taking proactive steps toward prevention, individuals can significantly reduce their risk of developing this life-altering condition. Lifestyle modifications, alongside regular medical check-ups, form the cornerstone of kidney disease prevention and overall kidney health.

Stages of Kidney Disease

Chronic Kidney Disease (CKD) progresses through five stages, with each stage reflecting a decline in kidney function. The progression is measured by the glomerular filtration rate (GFR), which estimates how much blood is filtered by the glomeruli (tiny filters in the kidneys) per minute. The stages of CKD are also characterized by the presence of kidney damage indicators, such as protein in the urine (proteinuria) or physical damage to the kidneys observable through imaging tests. Understanding these stages helps in managing the disease and planning treatment strategies.

Stage 1: Kidney Damage with Normal or High GFR (GFR ≥ 90 mL/min/1.73 m²)

In the earliest stage of CKD, the kidneys have sustained damage but still function efficiently, with a glomerular filtration rate (GFR) of 90 mL/min per 1.73 m² or higher. This damage can be detected through markers such as proteinuria (the presence of excessive protein in the urine) or hematuria (blood in the urine), abnormalities found via imaging tests (like ultrasounds or CT scans), or through biopsy results showing kidney tissue damage. Often, there are no noticeable symptoms at this stage, making early detection typically incidental through tests conducted for other reasons. Intervention strategies focus on identifying and managing the underlying causes of kidney damage, such as hypertension or diabetes, to prevent further decline in kidney function.

Stage 2: Mild Loss of Kidney Function (GFR 60-89 mL/min/1.73 m²)

Stage 2 CKD is marked by a mild reduction in kidney function, with GFR levels falling between 60 and 89 mL/min per 1.73 m². Similar to stage 1, symptoms might not be evident, and the presence of CKD is often identified through continued monitoring of kidney damage markers. At this stage, the emphasis is on slowing disease progression through the management of conditions that can cause further kidney damage, alongside lifestyle modifications such as

18

dietary changes, exercise, and smoking cessation. Monitoring blood pressure and blood sugar levels becomes increasingly important to address the primary causes of kidney stress.

Stage 3: Moderate Loss of Kidney Function (GFR 30-59 mL/min/1.73 m²)

Stage 3 CKD signifies a moderate decrease in kidney function, divided into sub-stages 3A (GFR 45-59 mL/min) and 3B (GFR 30-44 mL/min). This stage may bring more noticeable symptoms, including swelling (edema) in extremities, back pain, and changes in urination patterns (frequency, color, or consistency). Fatigue and weakness are common due to anemia, a result of the kidneys' diminished ability to produce erythropoietin, a hormone that stimulates red blood cell production. Management includes more aggressive measures to control blood pressure and blood sugar, dietary restrictions to ease the kidneys' workload, and possibly the introduction of medications to treat anemia and other arising complications.

Stage 4: Severe Loss of Kidney Function (GFR 15-29 mL/min/1.73 m²)

With a GFR of 15 to 29 mL/min per 1.73 m², stage 4 CKD indicates a severe reduction in kidney function. Symptoms become more pronounced, including significant fatigue from anemia, difficulty in concentrating, numbness or tingling in the extremities due to nerve damage, and disturbances in sleep patterns. Fluid retention can lead to hypertension and pulmonary edema, necessitating urgent medical interventions. This stage requires extensive planning for renal replacement therapy (RRT) such as dialysis or preparation for kidney transplantation, as well as managing cardiovascular risk factors to prevent heart disease, a common complication of advanced CKD.

Stage 5: Kidney Failure (GFR <15 mL/min/1.73 m²) or End-Stage Renal Disease (ESRD)

The final stage of CKD, stage 5, is characterized by kidney failure with a GFR of less than 15 mL/min per 1.73 m², signaling that the kidneys can no longer sustain life without intervention. Symptoms at this stage are severe and encompass a range of systemic effects including nausea, vomiting, a significant decrease in appetite leading to malnutrition, cognitive impairments, and fluid overload manifesting as swelling and shortness of breath. Treatment involves either dialysis, which artificially removes waste products and excess fluid from the blood, or a kidney transplant, which offers a chance at regaining normal kidney function. At this stage, comprehensive care is vital, addressing not only the physical aspects of the disease but also offering psychological and social support to patients and their families navigating these challenges.

Identifying the stage of CKD is critical for tailoring treatment approaches to individual needs, aiming to slow disease progression, manage symptoms, and maintain the highest possible quality of life. Each stage brings different challenges and requires adjustments in treatment and lifestyle, emphasizing the importance of close monitoring and collaboration between patients and healthcare teams.

Diagnosis and Tests

The diagnosis of kidney disease involves a combination of blood tests, urine tests, and imaging studies to assess kidney function, identify damage, and determine the underlying cause. This comprehensive approach helps healthcare providers diagnose kidney disease accurately and tailor treatment to the individual's needs. Here's what to expect during the diagnostic process and how to interpret test results.

Blood Tests

Serum Creatinine: The concentration of creatinine in the blood is a critical indicator of kidney function. Creatinine is a byproduct of muscle metabolism, typically filtered out by the kidneys. Elevated serum creatinine levels suggest that the kidneys are not filtering effectively. However, since creatinine levels can vary based on age, race, gender, and body size, they're used in conjunction with other tests to assess kidney function.

Glomerular Filtration Rate (GFR): The GFR is the gold standard for determining the stage of kidney disease. It measures the rate at which the kidneys filter blood, calculated from the serum creatinine level, age, body size, gender, and race. A GFR under 60 mL/min/1.73 m² for three months or longer indicates chronic kidney disease (CKD). The GFR not only confirms the presence of kidney disease but also helps in staging the disease, which is crucial for management and prognosis.

Blood Urea Nitrogen (BUN): Urea nitrogen is another waste product processed by the kidneys, originating from the breakdown of protein in foods. A high BUN level can indicate kidney dysfunction, though it's also influenced by factors such as dehydration, a high protein diet, and certain medications, making it less specific than GFR for kidney function.

Urine Tests

Urinalysis: This comprehensive test examines the physical, chemical, and microscopic aspects of urine. It can detect abnormalities like protein (proteinuria), blood (hematuria), white blood cells (indicative of infection), and sugar (a sign of diabetes). The persistent presence of protein or blood in the urine is a strong indicator of kidney damage.

Albumin-to-Creatinine Ratio (ACR): This test measures the ratio of albumin, a type of protein, to creatinine in a urine sample. It's especially useful for early detection of kidney damage in people with risk factors like diabetes or hypertension. An ACR higher than 30 mg/g is considered abnormal and suggests the presence of kidney disease.

Imaging Studies

Ultrasound: Kidney ultrasounds create images using sound waves, revealing the kidneys' size, shape, and position. It can detect masses, cysts, obstructions, and other structural abnormalities. Ultrasound is non-invasive and widely used in evaluating kidney disease.

CT Scan: A computed tomography (CT) scan offers detailed cross-sectional images of the kidneys, utilizing X-rays. It can identify stones, tumors, cysts, and other structural or vascular abnormalities. Contrast material is sometimes used to enhance visibility, though it may be contraindicated in severe CKD due to the risk of worsening kidney function.

MRI: Magnetic resonance imaging (MRI) provides high-resolution images of the kidneys and surrounding structures without using X-rays. It's particularly valuable for visualizing renal blood vessels and assessing complex kidney and urinary tract anomalies. Like CT scans, MRI may involve contrast agents, which require careful consideration in patients with kidney disease.

Kidney Biopsy

A biopsy is a definitive diagnostic procedure that involves removing a small sample of kidney tissue for microscopic examination. It's particularly helpful when the cause of kidney disease is unclear or when specific kidney disorders are suspected. A biopsy can diagnose conditions like glomerulonephritis, interstitial nephritis, and polycystic kidney disease, providing information on the extent of damage and guiding treatment.

Interpreting Test Results

Interpreting the results of these tests requires a comprehensive understanding of the patient's overall health, symptoms, and risk factors. Elevated serum creatinine and BUN levels, reduced GFR, and abnormalities in urine tests such as proteinuria and hematuria are key indicators of kidney dysfunction. Imaging studies can pinpoint structural causes of kidney problems, while a biopsy provides microscopic details about kidney damage.

Diagnosing kidney disease is a complex process that relies on a combination of tests. Continuous monitoring and periodic reevaluation are essential, especially for individuals at risk of CKD or those already diagnosed, to manage the condition effectively and mitigate progression. Collaboration between patients and healthcare providers is crucial for interpreting test results accurately and implementing an effective treatment plan.

Common Myths and Misconceptions

Kidney disease is surrounded by numerous myths and misconceptions that can hinder effective management and treatment. Dispelling these myths is crucial for fostering a better understanding of the condition, its impact, and the available treatment options. Here, we address some common myths and provide evidence-based information to correct misinformation.

Myth 1: Kidney Disease is Rare

Reality: Kidney disease is more common than many people think. Millions of people worldwide live with chronic kidney disease (CKD), and many are at risk due to underlying conditions such as diabetes and high blood pressure. The National Kidney Foundation estimates that 1 in 3 American adults is at risk for kidney disease, underscoring its prevalence.

Myth 2: Kidney Disease is Immediately Symptomatic

Reality: Kidney disease often progresses silently, without symptoms until it reaches an advanced stage. Early stages of CKD may not present any signs, making regular screening critical, especially for those at higher risk. Recognizing risk factors and undergoing periodic kidney function tests can lead to early detection and management.

Myth 3: Drinking Lots of Water Can Cure Kidney Disease

Reality: While staying hydrated is important for maintaining kidney health, drinking excessive amounts of water cannot cure kidney disease. Proper hydration helps the kidneys clear sodium, urea, and toxins from the body, which can reduce the risk of developing chronic kidney disease. However, once kidney damage is present, hydration alone is not a cure and must be accompanied by appropriate medical treatment.

Myth 4: Kidney Damage is Always Permanent

Reality: Not all kidney damage is irreversible. Acute kidney injury (AKI), for example, can sometimes be reversed if treated promptly and effectively. However, chronic kidney disease (CKD) involves more permanent damage that cannot be entirely reversed, though its progression can often be slowed with proper management.

Myth 5: Only Older People Get Kidney Disease

Reality: Kidney disease can affect individuals of all ages, including children. While the risk increases with age, particularly due to the higher prevalence of diabetes and high blood pressure in older adults, CKD can result from a variety of causes affecting people at any age, including genetic disorders, acute injury, or chronic conditions.

Myth 6: Kidney Disease Cannot Be Prevented

Reality: Many forms of kidney disease are preventable or can be delayed. Effective management of underlying conditions like diabetes and hypertension, maintaining a healthy lifestyle, avoiding excessive use of NSAIDs, and regular screening for those at risk can significantly reduce the likelihood of developing CKD.

Myth 7: If You Have Kidney Disease, You Will Definitely Need Dialysis

Reality: Not everyone with kidney disease will require dialysis. The treatment and management of CKD depend on the stage of the disease. Many people with CKD live for years without ever needing dialysis, managing their condition through medication, diet, lifestyle changes, and careful monitoring of their kidney function.

By debunking these myths, we can improve awareness and understanding of kidney disease, encouraging proactive health measures and timely, effective management. Knowledge is a powerful tool in preventing and managing CKD, helping those affected to lead healthier and more informed lives.

CHAPTER TWO: MANAGING KIDNEY DISEASE

Managing kidney disease is a multifaceted approach that requires careful consideration of diet, lifestyle modifications, precise medication management, vigilant health monitoring, and proactive handling of complications. This chapter guides you through the essential strategies to navigate the complexities of kidney disease, aiming to preserve kidney function, enhance quality of life, and prevent the condition from progressing. By integrating these key components into daily living, individuals can take active steps toward managing their kidney health effectively and mitigating the impact of the disease.

Dietary Management

Dietary management is a cornerstone of kidney disease treatment, requiring detailed attention to specific nutrients that impact kidney function. A nuanced approach to diet can help manage the disease's progression, alleviate symptoms, and enhance overall health. Here is an expanded overview of dietary adjustments for those managing kidney disease, emphasizing fluid intake, protein, potassium, phosphorus, and sodium, along with practical tips for implementing these changes.

Fluid Intake

The kidneys regulate fluid balance, but when their function is compromised, managing fluid intake becomes critical to prevent fluid overload, which can cause swelling, high blood pressure, and heart strain. The exact fluid requirement varies, influenced by residual kidney function, dialysis schedule (for those undergoing treatment), and daily urine output. Precise recommendations should be made by a healthcare provider, who can account for these factors and suggest an intake level that prevents dehydration while avoiding fluid retention.

Protein Management

While protein is an essential nutrient for bodily functions, including tissue repair and immune response, kidney disease necessitates moderation of protein consumption to reduce kidney workload. The dietary focus should be on high-quality proteins that provide essential amino acids with minimal waste production. Animal-based proteins (lean poultry, fish, and eggs) are considered high quality, but plant-based options (quinoa, soy products) are also excellent and can reduce the intake of saturated fats. The stage of kidney disease dictates the amount of protein required; early stages may not necessitate severe restrictions, whereas advanced stages or those on dialysis have different needs. A renal dietitian can create a protein plan that supports both your nutritional needs and kidney health.

Potassium Management

Potassium is vital for heart and muscle function. However, too much potassium can be dangerous for people with kidney disease, as impaired kidneys may not effectively remove it, leading to hyperkalemia, a condition that can cause heart rhythm disturbances. Dietary potassium management involves limiting high-potassium foods (such as bananas, avocados, potatoes, and spinach) and choosing lower-potassium alternatives (apples, berries, carrots, and green beans). Cooking methods like boiling can reduce the potassium content in vegetables. Regular monitoring of blood potassium levels guides dietary adjustments to maintain safe levels.

Phosphorus Management

Phosphorus plays a role in bone health, but CKD can lead to hyperphosphatemia, risking bone disease and cardiovascular issues. Many processed and convenience foods contain added phosphates, making label reading imperative. Natural phosphorus found in foods like dairy, nuts, and meats is absorbed more efficiently than added phosphates, so whole, unprocessed foods are preferable. Phosphorus binders may be prescribed to prevent absorption from the diet. Strategies include consuming meals lower in phosphorus and understanding the hidden sources in processed foods.

Sodium Management

Sodium intake affects blood pressure and fluid balance. Reducing sodium helps manage blood pressure and minimize edema and thirst, especially important for those on fluid restrictions. Seasoning foods with herbs and spices instead of salt, choosing fresh or frozen vegetables over canned ones, and avoiding processed meats can significantly reduce sodium intake. When grocery shopping, aim for foods labeled "low sodium" or "no salt added," and be cautious when eating out, as restaurant meals are often high in sodium.

Implementing Dietary Changes

- **Reading Food Labels:** Become adept at interpreting nutritional labels, paying close attention to servings per container and the amounts of sodium, potassium, phosphorus, and protein per serving.

- **Portion Control:** Familiarize yourself with serving sizes and use measuring cups or scales to ensure you're adhering to your dietary plan. Portion control is essential for managing the intake of critical nutrients.

- **Meal Planning and Preparation:** Planning meals in advance ensures dietary adherence and nutritional balance. Prepare meals at home to control ingredients, and when dining out, don't hesitate to request modifications that align with your dietary needs.

- **Consultation with a Renal Dietitian:** A dietitian specializing in kidney health can tailor your diet to your stage of kidney disease, lifestyle, and taste preferences, offering personalized advice, meal plans, and support.

- **Regular Monitoring and Adjustment:** Your dietary needs may change as kidney disease progresses or if you begin dialysis. Regular follow-ups with your healthcare team ensure your diet remains aligned with your current health status.

Dietary management in kidney disease is complex and personalized. Engaging with a healthcare team, especially a renal dietitian, is key to navigating these dietary changes effectively, ensuring they contribute positively to managing kidney disease and maintaining the best possible quality of life.

Lifestyle Changes

Managing kidney disease or slowing its progression involves a comprehensive approach to lifestyle modifications. These changes not only support kidney function but also contribute to overall well-being. Here's an in-depth look at essential lifestyle adjustments for individuals with kidney disease, including maintaining a healthy weight, regular exercise, smoking cessation, and stress management, with detailed tips for implementation.

Maintaining a Healthy Weight

Obesity is a significant risk factor for the development and progression of kidney disease, as it increases the likelihood of diabetes and hypertension, two leading causes of kidney damage. Achieving a healthy weight reduces the strain on the kidneys and helps control these risk factors.

Actionable Tips

- **Adopt a Nutrient-Rich Diet:** Focus on consuming a variety of fruits, vegetables, whole grains, and lean proteins. These foods are lower in calories and rich in nutrients, helping to manage weight effectively.
- **Practice Mindful Eating:** Heed signals of hunger and satisfaction to prevent overindulging. Consuming food slowly and free from distractions aids in identifying when you feel full.
- **Regular Monitoring:** Keep track of your weight through weekly check-ins and adjust your dietary intake and physical activity levels as needed.

Exercising Regularly

Physical activity is crucial for maintaining a healthy weight, reducing blood pressure, and decreasing the risk of cardiovascular diseases. It can also improve mood and reduce stress, which is beneficial for overall health.

Actionable Tips

- **Customize Your Exercise Plan:** Tailor your exercise routine to fit your current fitness level and kidney disease stage. Consult with a healthcare provider or a fitness professional who can help design a safe and effective program.

- **Incorporate Physical Activity into Daily Life:** Besides structured exercise, look for opportunities to be more active throughout the day, such as taking the stairs instead of the elevator, gardening, or walking during breaks.

- **Stay Consistent:** Maintaining a regular exercise routine is crucial for experiencing its advantages. Find a routine that fits into your schedule and lifestyle to maintain regular physical activity.

Quitting Smoking

Smoking is particularly harmful to those with kidney disease, as it further damages kidney tissue and exacerbates complications. Quitting smoking is one of the most significant steps you can take to protect your kidneys.

Actionable Tips

- **Use Available Resources:** Take advantage of quit-smoking resources, such as hotlines, online forums, and mobile apps designed to support individuals through the process.

- **Consider Medical Interventions:** Discuss with your healthcare provider about nicotine replacement therapies or prescription medications that can ease withdrawal symptoms and cravings.
- **Build a Support Network:** Engage family, and friends, or join support groups to gain encouragement and accountability during your quitting journey.

Managing Stress

Long-term stress can lead to high blood pressure and poor lifestyle choices, negatively impacting kidney health. Effective stress management is therefore crucial for individuals with kidney disease.

Actionable Tips

- **Regular Relaxation and Mindfulness Practices:** Engage in activities that promote relaxation, such as mindfulness meditation, progressive muscle relaxation, or guided imagery, to reduce stress.
- **Effective Time Management:** Organize your tasks and responsibilities to avoid last-minute rushes. Break down larger tasks into manageable steps and prioritize activities to reduce overwhelm.
- **Seek Professional Help if Needed:** If stress becomes overwhelming, consider seeking support from a mental health

professional who can offer coping strategies and therapeutic interventions.

Additional Lifestyle Tips

- **Hydration:** Proper hydration aids in kidney function, but those with advanced kidney disease may need to limit fluid intake. Follow your healthcare provider's recommendations regarding fluid consumption.
- **Alcohol Moderation:** If alcohol is consumed, it should be in moderation to avoid further kidney damage and complications with medications.
- **Sleep:** Ensure adequate sleep, as poor sleep can affect blood pressure, stress levels, and overall health. Strive to get 7-9 hours of restful sleep each night and set a consistent sleeping schedule.

Implementing these lifestyle changes requires commitment but can significantly improve kidney health and quality of life. It's essential to work closely with your healthcare team to tailor these recommendations to your specific needs and stage of kidney disease.

Medication Management

Effective medication management is fundamental in controlling kidney disease, mitigating its progression, and managing associated symptoms. It involves a nuanced understanding of various medications, their mechanisms, potential side effects, adherence strategies, and open communication with healthcare providers. Here's an expanded exploration of medication management for kidney disease.

Understanding Common Medications for Kidney Disease

Angiotensin-Converting Enzyme (ACE) Inhibitors and Angiotensin II Receptor Blockers (ARBs): These drugs lower blood pressure and decrease proteinuria, which can help slow kidney disease progression. They work by blocking pathways that tighten blood vessels, thereby improving blood flow and reducing the kidneys' workload. Commonly prescribed ACE inhibitors include enalapril and ramipril, while losartan and valsartan are frequently used ARBs. Monitoring for cough (more common with ACE inhibitors), hyperkalemia (high potassium levels), and renal function is crucial.

Diuretics: Different classes of diuretics act on various parts of the kidneys to promote fluid excretion, helping to manage blood pressure and fluid retention. Loop diuretics (furosemide), thiazide diuretics (hydrochlorothiazide), and potassium-sparing diuretics (spironolactone) are examples. Side effects may include dehydration, electrolyte imbalances, and increased urination frequency.

Phosphate Binders: These agents reduce phosphorus absorption from the diet, crucial for patients with advanced kidney disease to prevent bone and cardiovascular diseases. Calcium-based binders (calcium carbonate), non-calcium-based binders (sevelamer), and lanthanum carbonate are options. It's important to balance their use to avoid complications like hypercalcemia (high blood calcium levels) with calcium-based binders.

Erythropoiesis-Stimulating Agents (ESAs): ESAs treat anemia by mimicking the action of erythropoietin, a hormone produced by the kidneys that stimulates red blood cell production. They are beneficial for managing anemia-related fatigue and other symptoms. Risks include potential increases in blood pressure and the risk of thrombosis; thus, they must be used under careful supervision.

Calcium Channel Blockers: These medications relax blood vessels by blocking calcium's entry into the heart and blood vessel cells, reducing blood pressure and protecting the kidneys. Side effects can include lower limb edema, constipation, and dizziness.

Strategies for Medication Adherence

Adherence to medication regimes is vital for optimal outcomes in kidney disease management. Non-adherence can exacerbate disease progression, leading to avoidable complications.

Educational Interventions: Understanding the purpose and necessity of each medication can motivate adherence. Healthcare providers should explain why each medication is needed and how it contributes to managing kidney disease.

Simplifying Regimens: Whenever possible, simplifying the medication regimen by reducing the number of doses per day can enhance adherence.

Utilizing Technology: Mobile apps and digital reminders can provide timely prompts for medication intake, improving adherence rates.

Side Effect Management

Managing side effects is an integral part of medication management. For example, dietary adjustments can help manage hyperkalemia associated with ACE inhibitors or ARBs, while supplemental therapies can address anemia from ESAs. Regular monitoring through blood tests allows for early detection and management of side effects.

Medication management for kidney disease is complex and personalized, requiring a proactive approach from both patients and healthcare providers. Understanding the roles and risks of various medications, adhering to prescribed treatments, and maintaining open lines of communication with healthcare teams are key to managing kidney disease effectively. Through careful management, the impacts of kidney disease can be significantly mitigated, improving patient outcomes and quality of life.

Monitoring Your Health

Monitoring your health is a pivotal aspect of managing kidney disease effectively. It involves regular check-ups with healthcare providers, understanding lab results, and being vigilant about signs of disease progression. Active participation in monitoring your health can help in the early detection of complications, making timely adjustments to treatment plans, and potentially slowing the progression of kidney disease. Here's a detailed look at how to monitor your kidney health.

Regular Medical Check-ups

Regular check-ups are foundational for individuals managing kidney disease. These appointments allow your healthcare team to assess the progression of your disease, and the effectiveness of your treatment, and to adjust your care plan as needed.

- **Frequency and Schedule:** Depending on the stage of your kidney disease, your doctor will recommend a schedule for regular check-ups. Early stages may require bi-annual visits, whereas more advanced stages or those undergoing dialysis might necessitate monthly evaluations.

- **Comprehensive Evaluations:** During these appointments, expect a thorough review that may include physical examinations, blood pressure checks, and discussions about your diet, medication, and any symptoms you're experiencing.

Understanding and Tracking Lab Results

Being knowledgeable about your lab tests and what the results indicate is crucial in managing kidney disease.

- **Glomerular Filtration Rate (GFR):** This critical test measures your level of kidney function and determines your stage of kidney disease. A GFR below 60 mL/min/1.73 m² may indicate chronic kidney disease.

- **Urine Tests for Albumin:** The presence of albumin, a protein, in your urine, can be one of the first signs of kidney damage. The Albumin-to-Creatinine Ratio (ACR) quantifies this, helping to detect early kidney damage.

- **Serum Creatinine:** Elevated creatinine levels in your blood signal that your kidneys may not be functioning properly, as creatinine is a waste product that should be filtered out by your kidneys.

- **Blood Urea Nitrogen (BUN):** This test, which measures the amount of nitrogen in your blood that comes from the waste product urea, can provide additional insights into your kidney function.

Recognizing Signs of Progression

Staying vigilant about the signs and symptoms of kidney disease progression is critical. Key indicators include:

- **Swelling (Edema):** Look out for swelling in your legs, ankles, hands, or face, which might suggest fluid retention due to compromised kidney function.
- **Urination Changes:** Any changes in frequency, color, or the presence of foam or blood in your urine should be promptly discussed with your doctor.
- **Fatigue:** An unexplained increase in tiredness could be a sign of anemia associated with kidney disease.
- **Elevated Blood Pressure:** Difficulty in controlling blood pressure can indicate worsening kidney function.
- **Gastrointestinal Symptoms:** Nausea, vomiting, or a decrease in appetite could be signs of toxin buildup in your body.

Self-Monitoring Practices

Self-monitoring encompasses several practices that you can do at home to keep track of your health and provide valuable information to your healthcare team.

- **Blood Pressure Monitoring:** Regularly measuring your blood pressure at home can help ensure that hypertension, a common complication of kidney disease, is well-managed.

- **Weight Tracking:** Daily weight measurements can help identify fluid retention early. Sudden weight gain may indicate that your body is retaining more fluid than it should.
- **Symptom Journaling:** Keeping a diary of your daily symptoms, dietary intake, fluid intake, and physical activity can help identify patterns or triggers that may affect your kidney disease.

Effective monitoring of your health as you navigate kidney disease is a dynamic and continuous process. By understanding how to track and interpret changes in your condition, engaging in regular self-monitoring, and maintaining open lines of communication with your healthcare team, you can play an active role in managing your kidney disease and maintaining your quality of life.

Dealing with Complications

Managing the complications of kidney disease requires an in-depth understanding of how each condition affects the body and a comprehensive strategy to address these issues. Given the intricate relationship between kidney function and overall health, the complications of kidney disease—ranging from cardiovascular diseases to electrolyte imbalances—demand vigilant monitoring and proactive management. Here's an exploration into the prevention, early detection, and treatment of these complications.

Cardiovascular Diseases (CVD)

The interplay between kidney disease and cardiovascular health is complex. Kidney disease can lead to hypertension, atherosclerosis, heart failure, and arrhythmias due to the kidneys' role in fluid and electrolyte balance, blood pressure regulation, and erythropoietin production.

Prevention and Management

Integrated Cardio-Renal Approach: Managing CVD in kidney disease requires a coordinated approach that addresses both renal and cardiovascular health. This includes optimizing control of blood pressure and blood glucose levels, managing lipid levels, and addressing modifiable risk factors such as smoking and obesity.

Antihypertensive Therapy: A combination of lifestyle interventions and medications (ACE inhibitors, ARBs, beta-blockers, calcium channel blockers) tailored to the individual's needs can effectively manage hypertension. Regular monitoring is crucial to adjust treatment as kidney function changes.

Lifestyle Interventions: Dietary modifications to reduce sodium intake, increase intake of fruits and vegetables, regular physical activity, smoking cessation, and moderation of alcohol intake are foundational steps in reducing cardiovascular risk.

Anemia

Anemia arises when the kidneys fail to produce sufficient erythropoietin, leading to decreased red blood cell production. Chronic anemia can exacerbate cardiovascular problems, reduce oxygen delivery to tissues, and significantly impair quality of life.

Prevention and Management

Iron Supplementation: Both oral and intravenous iron supplements are used to treat iron deficiency, with the choice depending on the severity of anemia, kidney function, and response to treatment. Monitoring iron status through tests like ferritin and transferrin saturation helps guide therapy.

Erythropoiesis-Stimulating Agents (ESAs): These agents are critical for stimulating the bone marrow to produce red blood cells. Their use must be carefully balanced to avoid increasing the risk of thrombosis or worsening hypertension.

Nutritional Counseling: A dietitian can provide guidance on foods rich in iron, vitamin B12, and folate, which are important for red blood cell production.

Bone Disorders

Kidney disease disrupts the metabolism of calcium, phosphorus, and vitamin D, leading to bone mineralization defects, osteoporosis, and an increased risk of fractures. The management of bone health in kidney disease is multifaceted.

Prevention and Management

Monitoring and Management of Mineral Metabolism: Regular monitoring of serum calcium, phosphorus, PTH, and vitamin D levels is essential to guide the management of mineral and bone disorders. Treatments may include phosphate binders, calcimimetics, and vitamin D analogs or supplements.

Dietary Phosphorus Control: Dietary education focuses on limiting foods high in phosphorus (such as dairy products, nuts, and processed foods) and choosing foods with natural phosphorus, which is less absorbable.

Physical Activity: Weight-bearing exercises can help maintain bone density and strength, though individuals should consult with a healthcare provider to determine the appropriate level of activity.

Electrolyte Imbalances

Electrolyte imbalances, particularly of potassium, sodium, and calcium, are common in kidney disease and can have significant health implications, including cardiac arrhythmias, fluid retention, and neurological symptoms.

Targeted Intervention Strategies

Potassium Management: Dietary modification to limit high-potassium foods is often necessary. In some cases, medications like potassium binders or diuretics are prescribed to help maintain normal potassium levels.

Sodium and Fluid Balance: Recommendations typically include limiting sodium intake to control blood pressure and fluid balance. Diuretics may be used to manage fluid overload, but they must be carefully managed to avoid dehydration and electrolyte imbalances.

Calcium and Phosphorus Balance: Managing the delicate balance of calcium and phosphorus may involve dietary restrictions, phosphate binders, and vitamin D supplementation. The goal is to prevent hyperphosphatemia and its effects on bone health while avoiding hypercalcemia.

Proactive and Collaborative Care

Effectively dealing with the complications of kidney disease requires a proactive and collaborative care approach. Patients should work closely with their healthcare team—including nephrologists, dietitians, pharmacists, and nurses—to develop and maintain a comprehensive management plan. This plan should include regular monitoring of kidney function and related health indicators, personalized medication management, dietary counseling, and lifestyle modifications tailored to the individual's specific needs and stage of kidney disease.

By adopting a detailed and proactive strategy to monitor and manage the complications of kidney disease, individuals can mitigate the impact of these complications, enhancing their health outcomes and quality of life. Regular communication with healthcare providers, adherence to treatment plans, and lifestyle adjustments form the pillars of effective complication management in kidney disease.

CHAPTER THREE: TREATMENT OPTIONS

The journey through kidney disease treatment is marked by various paths, each tailored to the individual's condition and needs. This chapter explores the spectrum of treatment options, from conservative management, which focuses on diet and lifestyle modifications, to more invasive procedures like dialysis and kidney transplantation. It also delves into emerging treatments that offer new hope and discusses the role of holistic and alternative therapies in supporting kidney health. Together, these approaches provide a comprehensive framework for managing kidney disease, aiming to enhance quality of life and optimize outcomes.

Conservative Management

Conservative management of kidney disease emphasizes a multifaceted, non-pharmacological approach aimed at slowing disease progression, alleviating symptoms, and enhancing the patient's quality of life, particularly in the initial stages or for those for whom dialysis or transplantation isn't immediately considered. This strategy involves intricate dietary modifications, comprehensive lifestyle adjustments, and diligent monitoring. Here's an expanded discussion on each of these crucial elements.

Dietary Modifications

A carefully planned diet is pivotal in managing the workload on the kidneys and preventing the accumulation of waste products in the bloodstream.

- **Protein Consumption:** The body requires protein for growth and repair, but excessive intake can exacerbate kidney damage by increasing the kidneys' workload. The right balance depends on the individual's stage of kidney disease, with early stages possibly requiring normal intake and advanced stages necessitating significant reduction. A renal dietitian can tailor dietary advice, suggesting high-quality protein sources that minimize kidney strain.

- **Potassium and Phosphorus Management:** Impaired kidneys struggle to balance potassium and phosphorus, necessitating dietary adjustments to prevent dangerous complications like hyperkalemia, which affects heart rhythm, and hyperphosphatemia, which can lead to bone disease and calcification in the vessels. Patients are advised to limit or avoid high-potassium foods (such as bananas, oranges, and potatoes) and high-phosphorus foods (including dairy products, nuts, and certain meats), replacing them with safer alternatives.

- **Fluid Regulation:** As kidney disease progresses, the ability to manage fluid balance declines, risking fluid overload. Guidance on fluid intake varies significantly among individuals, factoring in residual kidney function and daily urine output. Excessive fluid can lead to high blood pressure, swelling, and heart issues, whereas too little intake can cause dehydration.

- **Sodium Intake:** Reducing sodium consumption is crucial for controlling blood pressure and minimizing swelling. Recommendations often involve consuming fresh, unprocessed foods over canned or processed items and creatively using herbs and spices for flavoring instead of salt.

Lifestyle Adjustments

Adopting a healthier lifestyle can significantly impact the management of kidney disease by supporting overall well-being and reducing risk factors associated with disease progression.

- **Physical Activity:** Engaging in regular physical activity, such as walking, cycling, or swimming, can improve cardiovascular health, aid in weight management, and enhance psychological well-being. The type and intensity of exercise should be customized to the individual's overall health and physical capabilities.

- **Smoking Cessation:** Smoking accelerates the progression of kidney disease and increases the risk of cardiovascular complications. Quitting smoking, often with the help of cessation programs or aids, is a critical component of conservative management.

- **Weight Management:** Achieving and maintaining a healthy weight through balanced nutrition and regular exercise can significantly reduce the pressure on the kidneys and mitigate risk factors like diabetes and hypertension.

- **Stress Management:** Chronic stress can have detrimental effects on health, potentially exacerbating kidney disease. Stress-reduction techniques such as mindfulness, yoga, and cognitive-behavioral strategies can be beneficial.

Diligent Monitoring

Regular monitoring allows for the early identification of changes in kidney function and the timely adjustment of management strategies.

- **Blood Pressure Monitoring:** Blood pressure is a vital sign for individuals with kidney disease, with strict control necessary to prevent further kidney damage and reduce cardiovascular risk.

- **Blood and Urine Tests:** Frequent laboratory tests, including serum creatinine, GFR, and urine albumin, provide insight into kidney function and disease progression. Understanding these results and their implications is essential for effective disease management.

- **Symptom Tracking:** Patients are encouraged to monitor and record any new or worsening symptoms, including changes in urination patterns, swelling, fatigue, or cardiovascular symptoms, and communicate these to their healthcare team promptly.

Conservative management requires a proactive and informed approach, with patients playing a central role in their care. Collaboration with a healthcare team, including nephrologists, dietitians, and nurses, ensures personalized and effective management. Through detailed dietary planning, lifestyle changes, and regular health monitoring, conservative management can significantly impact the course of kidney disease, preserving kidney function and maintaining the patient's quality of life.

Dialysis

Dialysis is a life-sustaining treatment for individuals with advanced kidney disease or kidney failure, where the kidneys can no longer perform their essential function of filtering waste products and excess fluids from the blood. Dialysis primarily comes in two varieties: hemodialysis and peritoneal dialysis. Each type has its processes, settings, and lifestyle considerations. Here's an in-depth exploration of both methods.

Hemodialysis

Process: Hemodialysis involves circulating the patient's blood outside the body through a machine equipped with a dialyzer, also known as an artificial kidney. The dialyzer filters out waste products, excess salts, and fluids from the blood, which is then returned to the patient's body. This process requires access to the patient's bloodstream, typically through a surgically created vein in the arm called an arteriovenous fistula, a graft, or a catheter.

What Patients Can Expect: Hemodialysis treatments are usually performed in a hospital or dialysis center, typically three times a week, with each session lasting about four hours. During treatment, patients are seated or lying down, and they can read, sleep, or watch TV. Some patients may experience side effects like low blood pressure, muscle cramps, or fatigue during or after treatment.

Managing Life with Hemodialysis: Adapting to life on hemodialysis requires scheduling flexibility, adherence to dietary and fluid intake restrictions, and regular travel to and from the dialysis center. It also demands strict management of medications and close monitoring of health indicators like blood pressure and weight.

Peritoneal Dialysis

Process: Peritoneal dialysis utilizes the patient's peritoneum (the lining of the abdominal cavity) as a natural filter. A dialysis solution is introduced into the abdomen through a permanently placed catheter. Waste products and excess fluids from the blood pass into the dialysis solution by osmosis and diffusion across the peritoneal membrane. After a dwell time, the fluid, now containing the filtered waste, is drained and replaced with a fresh solution.

What Patients Can Expect: Peritoneal dialysis can be performed at home, at work, or while traveling, offering more flexibility and independence than hemodialysis. There are two main types: Continuous Ambulatory Peritoneal Dialysis (CAPD), done manually four to five times a day; and Automated Peritoneal Dialysis (APD), performed at night using a machine. Patients need to maintain a sterile environment to prevent infections and are trained on how to perform exchanges.

Managing Life with Peritoneal Dialysis: Living with peritoneal dialysis involves daily treatment, which can be more accommodating to a patient's lifestyle compared to the fixed schedule of hemodialysis. Patients must monitor their catheter site for signs of infection and adhere to dietary recommendations, although these may be less restrictive than those for hemodialysis.

General Considerations for Dialysis

Diet and Fluid Intake: Both dialysis modalities necessitate meticulous dietary planning to balance electrolyte levels and prevent fluid retention. Collaboration with renal dietitians is invaluable in customizing nutritional strategies to accommodate individual health needs and treatment goals.

Emotional and Social Support: Adjusting to dialysis entails confronting emotional and social challenges, making support from healthcare providers, mental health counselors, and peer groups indispensable. These resources provide a coping mechanism, offering solace and guidance through shared experiences.

Physical Activity: Patients are encouraged to stay as active as possible, adapting activities to their energy levels and treatment schedules. Exercise can improve overall health, muscle function, and mood.

Employment and Travel: Many individuals on dialysis continue to work, attend school, and travel. Planning and coordination with the healthcare team are essential to accommodate treatment schedules and ensure that dialysis services are available when traveling.

Dialysis represents a significant adjustment in the lives of those with kidney failure, necessitating comprehensive medical care, lifestyle modifications, and emotional support. Through personalized treatment planning, education, and the support of a dedicated healthcare team, individuals on dialysis can manage their condition and maintain a fulfilling life.

Kidney Transplantation

Kidney transplantation stands as a beacon of hope for individuals battling end-stage renal disease (ESRD) or severe kidney failure, offering not just a treatment but a potential pathway to a life liberated from the constraints of dialysis. This procedure, while complex, is a testament to modern medicine's ability to significantly alter the course of chronic illnesses, providing patients with an opportunity to embrace a semblance of normalcy. Delving deeper into the transplantation process reveals its intricate nature, from evaluating eligibility to navigating post-transplant life.

Eligibility Assessment

The journey to a kidney transplant begins with a meticulous evaluation to determine a patient's suitability for this life-altering procedure. This assessment is multifaceted:

Comprehensive Health Evaluation: A detailed examination assesses not just kidney function but also the patient's cardiovascular health, cancer risk, and susceptibility to infections, ensuring they are strong enough to undergo surgery and handle post-operative care.

Psychosocial Assessment: Equally crucial is evaluating the patient's psychological readiness, social support systems, and their capacity to comply with a rigorous post-transplant medication and care regimen. This holistic assessment aims to ensure that patients are not only medically but also mentally and socially prepared for the transplantation and its aftermath.

Identifying a Compatible Donor

Identifying a suitable kidney donor is a pivotal step in the transplant process, involving:

Living Donors: The search often begins within the patient's circle but can extend to altruistic strangers. Living donors undergo a rigorous screening process to ensure they can safely donate a kidney, with considerations for their long-term health and the immediate benefit to the recipient. The advantages of living donations include shorter wait times and often better post-transplant outcomes due to the optimal health of the donor and organ.

Deceased Donors: Organs from deceased donors are allocated through a regulated system that prioritizes matches based on medical urgency, compatibility, and other ethical criteria. Despite the life-saving potential of these organs, the waiting time can be extensive, underscoring the critical need for organ donation awareness and registration.

Compatibility testing involves a series of sophisticated blood tests to ensure the donor and recipient are immunologically compatible, minimizing the risk of organ rejection.

The Transplant Procedure

Performed under general anesthesia, kidney transplant surgery is both a marvel of precision and a testament to medical advancement. The donated kidney is strategically placed in the recipient's lower abdomen, where its artery and vein are connected to existing blood vessels, and the ureter is linked to the bladder. This placement allows the new kidney to effectively filter blood and produce urine, marking the beginning of the recipient's post-transplant journey.

Navigating Post-Transplant Care

The post-transplant period is critical, necessitating vigilant care to ensure the transplant's success:

Immunosuppressive Therapy: The cornerstone of post-transplant care, this medication regimen is meticulously calibrated to prevent the immune system from attacking the new organ while balancing the risk of side effects and infections. Lifelong adherence to these medications is non-negotiable for transplant survival.

Holistic Health Management: Beyond medication, post-transplant care emphasizes a balanced diet, regular physical activity, and infection prevention. Patients are encouraged to adopt lifestyle changes that bolster their overall health and support the functioning of the transplanted organ.

Ongoing Monitoring and Support: Regular follow-up visits with the transplant team are essential to monitor organ function, adjust medications, and address any complications. Psychological support through counseling and support groups plays a vital role in helping patients and their families adapt to the changes and challenges post-transplant.

Kidney transplantation is more than a medical procedure; it's a journey that requires resilience, adherence, and an unwavering commitment to health and wellness. The success of this journey hinges on a collaborative effort among patients, healthcare providers, and the support of loved ones, offering a renewed chance at life for those with ESRD. Through careful patient selection, the generosity of donors, and the dedication of medical professionals, transplantation continues to be a critical, life-saving endeavor that embodies the pinnacle of therapeutic intervention in nephrology.

Emerging Treatments

The realm of kidney disease treatment is on the cusp of revolutionary advancements, propelled by cutting-edge research and technological innovation. These developments not only aim to refine and augment the efficacy of existing treatments but also explore previously untapped avenues that could fundamentally alter the therapeutic landscape for chronic kidney disease (CKD) and end-stage renal disease (ESRD). From pioneering pharmacological treatments to the nascent field of regenerative medicine and transformative dialysis technologies, here's a more detailed exploration of the emerging treatments reshaping kidney disease management.

Advanced Pharmacological Treatments

The pharmacological frontier is witnessing the introduction of novel medications designed to address the complex mechanisms underlying kidney disease, especially in patients with comorbid conditions such as diabetes.

SGLT2 Inhibitors: Sodium-glucose cotransporter-2 (SGLT2) inhibitors, such as empagliflozin and dapagliflozin, have transcended their initial role as antidiabetic agents to emerge as potent tools in combating CKD. Clinical trials have demonstrated their capacity to significantly reduce the risk of CKD progression, cardiovascular events, and hospitalization for heart failure in patients with type 2 diabetes by improving glycemic control, promoting weight loss, and lowering blood pressure, thereby alleviating the burden on the kidneys.

GLP-1 Receptor Agonists: Another class of drugs, glucagon-like peptide-1 (GLP-1) receptor agonists, initially used to treat type 2 diabetes, has shown promise in protecting kidney function. These medications enhance insulin secretion, suppress glucagon release, and may confer renal benefits by reducing inflammation and fibrosis in the kidneys.

Non-Steroidal Mineralocorticoid Receptor Antagonists (MRAs): The development of non-steroidal MRAs like finerenone offers a novel approach to mitigating CKD progression and cardiovascular risk without the pronounced hyperkalemia risk associated with earlier MRAs. By selectively blocking the harmful effects of aldosterone, these drugs can slow CKD progression and reduce cardiovascular mortality.

Breakthroughs in Regenerative Medicine

Regenerative medicine, particularly through stem cell therapy, offers unprecedented potential in repairing damaged kidney tissue and, eventually, in creating bioengineered organs for transplantation.

Mesenchymal Stem Cells (MSCs): The exploration into MSCs for their therapeutic potential in AKI and CKD is driven by their anti-inflammatory and tissue-regenerative properties. Ongoing clinical trials are evaluating the safety and efficacy of MSC therapies in modulating immune responses, promoting the repair of renal tissue, and restoring kidney function.

Kidney Organoids and Bioengineering: Advancements in stem cell biology have enabled the creation of kidney organoids, miniature, simplified versions of kidneys produced in vitro from pluripotent stem cells. These organoids hold promise for drug discovery, disease modeling, and the future of organ transplantation, potentially paving the way for bioengineered kidneys tailored to individual patients, thereby circumventing the challenges of donor organ shortages and immune rejection.

Dialysis Technology Innovation

Innovations in dialysis technology aim to enhance patient autonomy, improve treatment outcomes, and more closely replicate kidney functions.

Wearable Dialysis Devices: The concept of wearable artificial kidneys (WAK) is being explored to enable continuous, ambulatory dialysis, mimicking the kidney's natural function more closely than traditional dialysis methods. These devices aim to liberate patients from the constraints of fixed-time dialysis sessions, offering a more flexible and lifestyle-congruent treatment modality.

Bioartificial Kidneys: The development of bioartificial kidneys combines cellular therapy with microengineering to create devices that could one day replace the need for traditional dialysis and transplantation. These devices integrate renal cells with a bioreactor system, performing the essential functions of filtration, electrolyte balance, and waste removal, offering a holistic approach to renal replacement therapy.

The Horizon of Personalized Medicine

The advent of personalized medicine in kidney care involves tailoring treatment strategies to the individual genetic makeup, lifestyle, and disease pathology of each patient. Genetic and biomarker profiling enables healthcare providers to predict disease progression, tailor interventions, and monitor response to treatment with unparalleled precision.

The evolving landscape of kidney disease treatment heralds a future where management strategies are not only more effective and less invasive but also highly personalized. As these emerging treatments progress from clinical trials to standard care, they hold the promise of transforming the prognosis for individuals with CKD and ESRD, offering hope for improved quality of life and long-term outcomes.

Holistic and Alternative Therapies

The incorporation of holistic and alternative therapies into the realm of kidney health management represents a nuanced approach, aiming to enhance the well-being of individuals navigating the challenges of kidney disease. These therapies, spanning from herbal remedies to mind-body practices, offer a complementary pathway alongside conventional medical treatments. However, their integration demands a critical understanding of their efficacy, potential risks, and the overarching importance of a collaborative dialogue with healthcare professionals.

Herbal Remedies

Herbal supplements and natural remedies often allure patients with their traditional uses and perceived safety. However, the therapeutic landscape for kidney disease is complex, necessitating a cautious approach:

Herbal Diuretics and Kidney Function: Some herbs are touted for their diuretic properties, purportedly aiding in fluid regulation. Yet, their indiscriminate use in CKD can lead to electrolyte imbalances and potentially worsen kidney function.

Nephrotoxic Risks: The spectrum of herbal remedies includes plants such as Aristolochia, which have been implicated in causing severe kidney damage and urothelial cancers. Similarly, supplements like creatine, used for muscle building, can strain kidney function when used excessively.

Interaction with Standard Medications: The metabolic pathways involved in the breakdown and absorption of both herbal and conventional medicines can intersect, leading to decreased drug efficacy or enhanced toxicities. For instance, herbal supplements like garlic and ginkgo can increase the risk of bleeding when taken with anticoagulants.

Acupuncture

Acupuncture, with its roots in ancient medical traditions, has been explored for its potential to address symptoms of CKD such as chronic pain and fatigue. The practice involves:

Targeted Needle Insertion: By stimulating specific points, acupuncture aims to modulate the body's energy flow, or Qi, which can translate to symptom relief. However, the evidence supporting its efficacy varies, and needle insertion sites must be chosen with care, especially in patients with compromised skin integrity.

Considerations for ESRD Patients: Those with advanced kidney disease may have altered immune responses, making infection control paramount during acupuncture treatments.

Mind-Body Practices

The synergy between mental and physical health is the cornerstone of mind-body practices, which encompass:

Meditation and Stress Management: Techniques such as guided imagery, mindfulness meditation, and progressive muscle relaxation can significantly mitigate stress levels, which is particularly beneficial in managing hypertension, a common comorbidity in CKD.

Yoga and Tai Chi: These gentle exercises not only foster physical strength and flexibility but also contribute to mental well-being.

Their low-impact nature makes them suitable for individuals with varying degrees of kidney health, promoting circulation and reducing stress without overburdening the kidneys.

Navigating the Path with Caution

The journey through holistic and alternative therapies must be navigated with discernment and an evidence-based approach:

Collaborative Healthcare Dialogue: Open communication with nephrologists, pharmacists, and dietitians is essential to safely incorporate alternative therapies into kidney disease management. This collaborative effort ensures therapies complement rather than compromise standard treatment protocols.

Critical Evaluation of Therapies: Patients and healthcare providers together should critically assess the scientific merit and safety profile of alternative therapies, steering clear of those with unsubstantiated claims or known risks.

Adverse Effects and Monitoring: Vigilance in monitoring the impact of any new therapy on kidney function and overall health is imperative, with any adverse changes promptly communicated to the healthcare team.

In sum, while holistic and alternative therapies offer potential supportive benefits in the context of kidney disease, their integration into care plans requires a meticulously informed, cautious, and collaborative approach. This ensures that such therapies truly complement the broader objectives of enhancing patient well-being, managing disease symptoms, and supporting kidney health safely and effectively.

CHAPTER FOUR: LIVING WITH KIDNEY DISEASE

Living with kidney disease presents a multifaceted challenge that extends beyond physical health, encompassing emotional, psychological, financial, and social dimensions. This chapter delves into the critical support systems and strategies essential for navigating the complexities of kidney disease. From securing emotional and psychological support, understanding healthcare navigation, and addressing financial and legal considerations, to tapping into community resources, we explore avenues to enhance the quality of life for individuals affected by kidney disease, ensuring they are not alone in their journey.

Emotional and Psychological Support

The diagnosis of kidney disease often brings about a profound emotional upheaval, leading to a complex spectrum of feelings ranging from denial and anger to depression and anxiety. The chronic nature of the disease, coupled with the demands of treatment such as dialysis, can significantly impact one's mental health, sense of autonomy, and overall quality of life. Recognizing and addressing these psychological challenges is as crucial as managing the physical aspects of the disease.

Understanding the Emotional Toll

The emotional and psychological landscape for those with kidney disease is marked by several factors:

Chronic Uncertainty: Living with a chronic condition like kidney disease often means facing ongoing uncertainty about the future, including concerns about disease progression, treatment efficacy, and the potential need for dialysis or transplantation. This uncertainty can lead to chronic stress and anxiety, exacerbating the emotional toll of the disease.

Grief and Loss: Patients may experience grief over the loss of their health and the life they had before their diagnosis. This grieving process can involve anger, denial, bargaining, depression, and acceptance, similar to grieving the loss of a loved one.

Isolation and Social Withdrawal: The visible signs of treatment, dietary and fluid restrictions, and fatigue can make social interactions challenging, leading to feelings of isolation and loneliness. The fear of stigma or not wanting to burden others can further drive social withdrawal.

Coping Strategies

Developing coping mechanisms is essential for navigating the emotional challenges of kidney disease:

Seeking Knowledge: Understanding the ins and outs of kidney disease can empower patients, reduce feelings of helplessness, and foster a proactive attitude toward disease management. Educated patients are better equipped to participate in their care, ask informed questions, and make decisions that align with their values and goals.

Building a Support System: Establishing a robust support network, including family, friends, healthcare providers, and fellow patients, can provide a sense of belonging and community. Sharing experiences and feelings with others who understand can be incredibly validating and reduce feelings of isolation.

Support from Mental Health Experts: Turning to psychological wellness support, like therapy or counseling, arms people with approaches to reduce stress, lessen the impact of depression or anxiety, and manage the mental challenges stemming from chronic health issues. Cognitive-behavioral therapy (CBT), in particular, can be effective in changing negative thought patterns and improving emotional well-being.

Mental Health Care as a Priority

Integrating mental health care into the overall treatment plan for kidney disease is vital:

Routine Mental Health Screening: Regular screening for mental health conditions should be a standard part of care for individuals with kidney disease, allowing for early identification and intervention.

Tailored Psychological Interventions: Psychological interventions should be tailored to the individual's specific needs, considering the stage of the disease, the patient's circumstances, and their emotional response to their condition.

Psychoeducation: Providing patients and their families with information about the psychological aspects of kidney disease and available mental health resources can demystify the experience and encourage the seeking of support.

Resources and Support Networks

Leveraging available resources and joining support networks can significantly enhance emotional resilience:

Kidney Disease Support Groups: Both online and in-person support groups offer a platform for sharing experiences, tips, and emotional support, helping to reduce feelings of isolation.

Educational Resources: Organizations dedicated to kidney health often provide comprehensive educational materials, workshops, and seminars that address both the physical and emotional aspects of living with kidney disease.

Wellness Programs: Participating in wellness and mindfulness programs, such as meditation classes, yoga, or art therapy, can offer therapeutic outlets for stress relief and emotional expression.

Living with kidney disease is undeniably a multifaceted challenge that demands attention to both physical and emotional well-being. By acknowledging the psychological impact, seeking appropriate support, and utilizing coping strategies, individuals with kidney disease can navigate their journey with greater resilience, maintaining their mental health and enhancing their quality of life amidst the challenges posed by their condition.

Navigating Healthcare

Navigating the healthcare landscape with kidney disease necessitates a proactive and informed approach. This involves not just passive participation but active engagement in your healthcare journey. Effective communication with healthcare providers, robust self-advocacy, and a thorough understanding of patient rights are pivotal to securing optimal care and treatment outcomes. Here is an expanded guide on how to navigate healthcare effectively when living with kidney disease.

Effective Communication with Healthcare Providers

The relationship between patients and their healthcare providers is at the heart of effective disease management. Here's how to optimize this dynamic:

Document and Share Your Health History: Keep a detailed record of your health history, including previous treatments, hospitalizations, allergies, and reactions to medications. Sharing this information with your healthcare team ensures a comprehensive understanding of your condition.

Active Participation in Appointments: Approach each appointment as an active participant. This means asking questions, expressing concerns, and discussing treatment preferences. Consider bringing a family member or friend to appointments for support and to help remember the information discussed.

Feedback on Treatment Plans: Provide feedback on your treatment plan, including any side effects you're experiencing or difficulties with adherence. This feedback is invaluable for tailoring your care to your needs.

Utilize Technology: Many healthcare systems offer patient portals where you can access your medical records, and test results, and communicate with your healthcare team. Take advantage of these tools to stay informed and engaged in your care.

Mastering Self-Advocacy in Healthcare

Self-advocacy is crucial for ensuring your healthcare needs are met. Here's how to advocate effectively for yourself:

Develop a Healthcare Philosophy: Identify what you value in your care (e.g., a holistic approach, aggressive treatment of symptoms). Communicating this philosophy to your healthcare team helps align your care with your values.

Stay Informed: Use reputable sources to educate yourself about kidney disease, treatment options, and the latest research. This knowledge empowers you to engage in meaningful discussions about your care.

Establish Clear Communication: Express your needs, preferences, and concerns clearly to your healthcare providers. If you feel your concerns are not being addressed, don't hesitate to reiterate them or seek additional opinions.

Network with Other Patients: Connecting with others who have kidney disease can provide insights into navigating the healthcare system and advocating for yourself. Support groups and online forums are valuable resources for sharing experiences and advice.

Understanding Patient Rights

Being knowledgeable about your rights as a patient is fundamental. Here's what you need to know:

Informed Consent: You have the right to receive clear, understandable information about your treatment options, including the potential risks and benefits, to make informed decisions about your care.

Right to Privacy: The Health Insurance Portability and Accountability Act (HIPAA) protects your medical information. Understanding your privacy rights helps ensure your information is handled appropriately.

Access to Your Medical Records: Knowing how to access your medical records empowers you to review your treatment history, understand your condition better, and share this information with any new healthcare providers.

Navigating Insurance and Financial Assistance: Understanding your insurance coverage, including what treatments and medications are covered, is crucial. For uncovered expenses, explore patient assistance programs offered by pharmaceutical companies, non-profit organizations, and government agencies.

Complaints and Appeals Process: Familiarize yourself with the process for filing complaints or appeals within your healthcare system and insurance company. Knowing how to navigate these processes ensures that your voice is heard and your care needs are addressed.

Navigating healthcare with kidney disease requires a multifaceted strategy that emphasizes clear communication, self-advocacy, and an in-depth understanding of patient rights. By adopting these strategies, you empower yourself to take an active role in your healthcare, ensuring that your treatment aligns with your needs, preferences, and values, thereby enhancing your overall quality of life and health outcomes.

Financial and Legal Considerations

Managing kidney disease encompasses navigating through a complex maze of financial and legal considerations that extend far beyond the immediate realm of medical treatments. The financial implications of long-term care, medications, and the potential for income loss due to illness can pose daunting challenges. Equally important are the legal aspects related to employment, disability rights, and insurance entitlements. This section aims to provide comprehensive insights into effectively managing these dimensions, ensuring patients and their families are well-equipped to handle the financial and legal intricacies of kidney disease treatment.

Navigating Insurance

Insurance coverage is a critical factor in the financial management of kidney disease, significantly affecting access to necessary treatments and medications.

Policy Review: It's imperative to thoroughly review your insurance policy, understanding not just the headline benefits but also the fine print that outlines coverage limits, exclusions, and the specifics of coverage for kidney disease treatments, including dialysis, kidney transplantation, and associated medications.

Pre-authorization and Appeals: Familiarize yourself with your insurance provider's pre-authorization process, which is a prerequisite for many treatments and procedures. In the event of a denial, the appeals process becomes crucial. This might involve compiling comprehensive medical evidence and securing detailed support from your healthcare team to contest the insurer's decision.

Supplemental Insurance Options: For those covered under Medicare or similar programs, exploring supplemental insurance (like Medigap) can provide additional coverage for out-of-pocket expenses not covered by primary insurance. This additional layer of coverage can mitigate the financial burden of copayments, deductibles, and coinsurance.

Maximizing Patient Assistance Programs

Patient assistance programs can provide a lifeline by offering financial aid or access to medications at reduced costs or for free.

Pharmaceutical Company Programs: These programs often target patients based on financial need or lack of adequate insurance coverage. Eligibility criteria can vary widely, making it essential to research and apply to programs for which you may qualify.

Support from Non-Profit Organizations: Entities like the American Kidney Fund (AKF) play a pivotal role in providing financial assistance and support services to kidney disease patients. These programs can help cover the costs of treatment, medications, and even insurance premiums.

Utilizing Government Assistance: Beyond Medicaid, patients should explore all available government assistance programs, including those offered by the Social Security Administration (SSA) for disability benefits. These programs can provide crucial financial support and healthcare coverage for eligible individuals.

Understanding Legal Rights and Protections

Legal protections are in place to support individuals with kidney disease in maintaining their employment and accessing necessary accommodations or benefits.

Americans with Disabilities Act (ADA): This act safeguards individuals with chronic conditions like kidney disease from workplace discrimination and mandates reasonable accommodations to enable them to perform their jobs, including modified schedules or adjustments to work environments.

Family and Medical Leave Act (FMLA): The FMLA provides eligible employees with the right to take unpaid, job-protected leave for serious health conditions, offering a crucial buffer for those needing time off for treatment without fear of losing their employment.

Social Security Disability Insurance (SSDI): For individuals unable to work due to the severity of their kidney disease, SSDI offers financial assistance. The application process is stringent, requiring detailed proof of the disability and its impact on employment capabilities.

Financial Planning and Management

Effective financial management involves more than just budgeting; it requires a strategic approach to navigate the costs associated with kidney disease treatment.

Budgeting: A detailed budget should account for all medical and related expenses, incorporating strategies for managing out-of-pocket costs and maximizing insurance benefits.

Seeking Financial Counseling: Many healthcare facilities provide financial counseling services to help patients navigate their insurance benefits, understand their medical bills, and identify potential assistance programs.

Legal Consultation: For complex situations, such as disputes over insurance coverage or applying for disability benefits, legal consultation with experts in healthcare or disability law can provide invaluable guidance and support.

Navigating the financial and legal landscapes of kidney disease treatment is a multifaceted challenge that demands diligent research, proactive management, and strategic planning. Armed with a comprehensive understanding of insurance intricacies, patient assistance options, legal rights, and financial management strategies, patients and their families can mitigate the impact of kidney disease, ensuring a focus on health and well-being amidst these challenges.

Community and Resources

The journey through kidney disease can often feel isolating, but finding community and tapping into a wide array of resources can significantly lighten the burden. Community support plays a pivotal role in coping with the emotional, psychological, and practical challenges of kidney disease. It provides a platform for sharing experiences, gaining valuable insights, and accessing a wealth of information and assistance. Here's a detailed exploration of how individuals living with kidney disease can connect with support groups, engage in online forums, and involve themselves with kidney disease advocacy organizations.

The Power of Support Groups

Support groups bring together individuals facing similar challenges, offering a sense of belonging and understanding that is hard to find elsewhere. These groups can be found through:

- **Hospitals and Treatment Centers:** Many healthcare facilities host support groups for patients with kidney disease and their families. These groups often meet regularly, providing a space to share personal experiences, discuss treatment options, and offer emotional support.

- **Non-Profit Organizations:** Organizations dedicated to kidney health, such as the National Kidney Foundation (NKF) and the American Kidney Fund (AKF), often organize support groups and community events. These groups can be invaluable resources for education, advocacy, and support.

- **Specialized Support Services:** Some organizations offer support groups for specific segments of the kidney disease community, such as patients on dialysis, kidney transplant recipients, or those living with a particular type of kidney disease. These specialized groups can provide targeted advice and support.

Engaging with Online Forums and Social Media

The digital age has facilitated the creation of vibrant online communities where individuals can seek support, share experiences, and access information from anywhere in the world. Online forums and social media platforms offer:

- **Immediate Access to Community:** Online forums dedicated to kidney disease, such as those hosted on the websites of kidney health organizations or social media groups, provide a platform for real-time communication and support.

- **Anonymity and Privacy:** For those who prefer to seek advice and share experiences without revealing their identity, online forums can offer a level of anonymity and privacy not always available in face-to-face support groups.

- **Diverse Perspectives:** Online communities often include members from various geographical locations, offering a wide range of experiences and insights that can help navigate the complexities of kidney disease.

Involvement with Kidney Disease Advocacy Organizations

Kidney disease advocacy organizations play a crucial role in raising awareness, funding research, and advocating for policies that benefit the kidney disease community. Involvement with these organizations can provide opportunities to:

- **Access Educational Resources:** These organizations offer a wealth of information on kidney disease, treatment options, living a healthy lifestyle with kidney disease, and more. Accessing these resources can empower patients and their families with knowledge.

- **Participate in Events and Fundraisers:** Many advocacy organizations host events, workshops, and fundraisers that individuals can participate in. These events not only raise awareness and funds for kidney disease but also provide opportunities for community building.

- **Advocate for Change:** Getting involved in advocacy efforts can give individuals a sense of purpose and the chance to contribute to meaningful change, whether by advocating for policy changes, participating in awareness campaigns, or volunteering.

Finding community and accessing resources are crucial steps in managing the challenges of kidney disease. Support groups, online forums, and involvement with kidney disease advocacy organizations offer avenues for connection, education, and empowerment. These resources not only provide emotional and practical support but also foster a sense of community and belonging, reminding individuals that they are not alone on their journey with kidney disease.

Quality of Life

Enhancing the quality of life while managing kidney disease is a comprehensive endeavor that goes beyond mere medical treatment. It encompasses nurturing mental, emotional, and social well-being, alongside maintaining physical health. This holistic approach aims not just at longevity but at enriching life's quality despite the disease's challenges. Here's a deeper dive into strategies for living well with kidney disease.

Staying Physically Active

Physical activity is a cornerstone of maintaining and improving the quality of life for those with kidney disease. It bolsters physical health while providing mental and emotional benefits.

- **Tailored Exercise Plans:** Collaborating with healthcare professionals to create an exercise plan that respects your medical needs and limitations is crucial. This plan should consider factors like cardiovascular health, energy levels, and any dialysis-related considerations.
- **Diverse and Enjoyable Activities:** Incorporating a variety of activities can keep exercise engaging and reduce monotony. From low-impact sports and water aerobics to dance classes and

gentle stretching routines, finding activities you enjoy ensures consistency in staying active.

- **Gradual Progression:** Building up the intensity and duration of physical activities gradually helps prevent overexertion and minimizes the risk of injury. Celebrating small milestones can motivate continued effort and improvement.

Engaging in Hobbies and Interests

Engaging in hobbies and interests provides a vital outlet for stress relief and personal expression, contributing significantly to overall well-being.

- **Creative Pursuits:** Creative activities such as drawing, writing, or playing music not only offer a means of expression but also can serve as therapeutic outlets, helping to process feelings and experiences related to living with kidney disease.

- **Learning and Development:** Pursuing new skills or knowledge areas through online courses, workshops, or community college classes can provide a sense of achievement and mental stimulation, countering feelings of stagnation or limitation imposed by the disease.

- **Adapting for Enjoyment:** Modifying how you engage in your favorite hobbies to accommodate any physical limitations is key. This might involve using ergonomic tools for gardening or setting up a comfortable workspace for crafting.

Maintaining Social Connections

Social support is integral to emotional health, offering a buffer against stress and a source of joy and companionship.

- **Proactive Communication:** Keeping open lines of communication with family and friends about your needs and experiences helps maintain strong relationships and ensures support when needed.

- **Expanding Networks:** Exploring new social circles through community classes, online groups, or volunteer work can enrich your social life and introduce you to people with shared interests or similar experiences.

- **Support System Diversification:** Balancing your support system to include healthcare professionals, close family, friends, and peers from support groups can provide a well-rounded network of emotional and practical support.

Prioritizing Mental Health

Addressing the psychological impacts of kidney disease is as important as managing its physical aspects.

- **Comprehensive Mental Health Care:** Regular consultations with a psychologist or psychiatrist familiar with chronic illness can help manage the mental health challenges of kidney disease, providing coping mechanisms and therapeutic interventions.

- **Mindfulness and Stress Reduction:** Engaging in mindfulness practices, yoga, or tai chi can enhance emotional regulation, reduce anxiety, and improve stress management, contributing to a more balanced mental state.

- **Education and Advocacy:** Empowering yourself through education about kidney disease and advocating for your needs and rights can foster a sense of control and agency, positively impacting mental health.

Enhancing the quality of life while living with kidney disease is an ongoing, dynamic process that requires attention to the body, mind, and spirit. By actively engaging in physical activities, pursuing hobbies, strengthening social bonds, and prioritizing mental health, individuals can navigate the complexities of kidney disease with resilience and positivity. This holistic approach not only addresses the multifaceted challenges of the condition but also opens avenues for fulfillment, joy, and a deeply meaningful life despite the constraints of chronic illness.

CONCLUSION

In closing this guide on navigating the complexities of kidney disease, it's essential to recognize the multifaceted nature of this condition. Beyond the realm of medical treatments, managing kidney disease demands a holistic approach that equally addresses the physical, emotional, and social facets of well-being. This guide has endeavored to arm you with a comprehensive understanding and the necessary tools to confidently tackle the challenges of kidney disease, advocating for a proactive and empowered stance in your healthcare journey.

Throughout this book, we've traversed the essential aspects of kidney disease, from grasping its early signs to exploring the spectrum of treatment options, including dialysis, transplantation, and the promising horizon of emerging therapies. We've emphasized the critical role of emotional and psychological support, outlined effective strategies for navigating the healthcare system, and discussed the financial and legal intricacies that accompany this condition.

Furthermore, we delved into ways to enrich your quality of life, highlighting the importance of staying active, indulging in hobbies, and fostering social connections. Each section was meticulously designed to highlight the significance of taking charge of your disease management and the empowerment that stems from being well-informed and actively involved in your care.

With the insights gleaned from this book, you are encouraged to take a dynamic role in your healthcare journey. The act of advocating for your health is paramount—initiate transparent conversations with your healthcare providers, pose questions, and undertake your research to ensure your treatment plan is tailored to your unique needs and aspirations. True empowerment is born from making informed healthcare decisions, championing your needs, and maintaining an optimistic perspective in the face of kidney disease challenges.

Let this guide serve as the foundation for a path of self-advocacy and empowerment. Absorb the knowledge imparted, apply the strategies discussed, and remember, that you are the most pivotal player in your healthcare team. Your involvement, curiosity, and decisions significantly influence your health outcomes and life quality.

To further bolster your journey with kidney disease, an array of resources stands ready to offer additional support, information, and a sense of community. Renowned organizations such as the National Kidney Foundation and the American Kidney Fund offer extensive resources, from educational content about kidney disease and its treatments to support programs designed for patients. Additionally, online forums and social media platforms provide spaces for individuals with kidney disease to share experiences, advice, and encouragement, fostering a supportive community of understanding and empathy.

As you forge ahead, navigating the intricacies of kidney disease, carry with you the knowledge that, equipped with the right information, a robust support network, and a proactive approach to your care, you can confront kidney disease with confidence and resilience. May this book not only serve as a guide but also as a steadfast companion on your journey, empowering you to advocate for your health and live your life to its fullest potential, despite the hurdles you may encounter.